# Essays on Mental Illness
*Real People, Real Life, Real Hope*
Expanded Version

compiled and edited by

Caroline S. Cooper

Copyright © 2019 by Caroline S. Cooper All rights reserved.

ISBN 9781985197442

Caroline S. Cooper
410 SE Brentwood Drive
Lee's Summit, MO 64063
caroline@ingodscorner.org
www.ingodscorner.org

No part of this publication may be reproduced, stored in a retrieval system or transmitted in any way by any means, electronic, mechanical, photocopy, recording or otherwise without the prior permission of the author except as provided by USA copyright law.

Scripture quotations marked "NASB" are taken from the Holy Bible, New American Standard Bible®, (NASB) Copyright © 1960, 1962, 1963, 1968, 1971, 1972, 1973, 1975, 1977, 1995 by The Lockman Foundation. Used by permission." (www.Lockman.org). As found in the Logos Bible study software program.

Scripture quotations marked "NIV" are taken from the Holy Bible, New International Version ®, Copyright © 1973, 1978, 1984 by International Bible Society. Used by permission of Zondervan Publishing House. All rights reserved. As found in the Logos Bible study software program.

Scripture quotations marked "NLT" are taken from the Holy Bible, New Living Translation, Copyright © 1996. Used by permission of Tyndale House Publishers, Inc. All rights reserved. As found in the Logos Bible study softwar program.

Scripture quotations marked "NKJV" are taken from the Holy Bible: The New King James Version. 1982. Nashville: Thomas Nelson. As found in the Logos Bible study software program.

Scripture quotations marked "KJV" are taken from the The Holy Bible, King James Version. New York: American Bible Society: 1999; Bartleby.com, 2000. www.bartleby.com/108/. As found in the Logos Bible study software program.

Scripture quotations marked "MSG" are taken from The Holy Bible, Holy Bible: The Message (the Bible in contemparary language). 2005. Colorado Springs, CO: NavPress. As found in the Logos Bible study software program.

This book contains information regarding mental health and recovery. It is provided with the understanding that the author is not engaged in individualized professional services. Professional therapy or medical treatment should be used when necessary for a person's behavioral and emotional well-being.

# Dedication

To family and friends of individuals learning
to cope with mental health challenges

To anyone embracing life to the fullest
while living with mental illness

*Your perseverance and courage are inspiring!*

---

# Important Note

This book contains stories from real people, sharing openly and honestly. Please be aware that some of the content may be disturbing and cause an individual to be triggered. *Please stop reading immediately if this happens and only return to that particular story if you believe you can remain composed for a healthy experience.*

I will keep you in my prayers, praying that God will give you hope and encouragement in your life situations as you read these essays.

# TABLE OF CONTENTS

**A Roller Coaster Life** ........................................................................ 3
    by Caroline S. Cooper

**Loosing Daddy** ................................................................................. 7
    by Jane Alexander

**I Am Not My Illness or My Trauma:** ................................................ 9
    by Susan M. Clabaugh

**A Comparison - Depression and a Man Lost at Sea** ..................... 13
    A Poetic Reflection by Kaitlyn Wallace

**Prayer and Psychiatry** .................................................................... 15
    by Zeta Combs Davidson

**Perseverance: A Way of Life** .......................................................... 19
    by Beth

**The Woman in the Mirror** ............................................................. 21
    by Tess

**Sleeping Free** .................................................................................. 27
    A Poem by Caroline S. Cooper

**Depression, Anxiety, Acceptance, Success** .................................. 29
    by Sara

**Anxious Thoughts Turn to Hope** ................................................... 33
    by Cindy Richardson

**Grief and Tears** ............................................................................... 41
    Poems by Cindy Richardson

**Jane's Journey** ................................................................................ 43
    by Jane Alexander

**"Keep Your Powder Dry"** ............................................................... 47
    by Bill

**Hopeless and Hopeful** ...................................................................53
  *Poems by Cindy Richardson*

**Cyclothymia** ..............................................................................55
  *by Judith Vander Wege*

**Hope for Depression Healing** ............................................61
  *Zeta Combs Davidson*

**From Prison to Purpose** .....................................................65
  *by Joshua Callahan*

**Surviving Home With my Mother** ....................................67
  *Stories and Poems by Rosie Maureen*

**Hold Me Jesus** ......................................................................75
  *Poems by Cindy Richardson*

**Who Am I?** ............................................................................77
  *by Caroline S. Cooper*

**Appendix I – Be an Encourager** ........................................79

**Appendix II – Resources** ....................................................83

**About the Author** ................................................................85

> But there was no need to be ashamed
> of tears, for tears bore witness that
> a man had the greatest of courage,
> the courage to suffer.
>
> Viktor E. Frankl
> *Man's Search for Meaning*

Essays on Mental Illness

# A Roller Coaster Life
*by Caroline S. Cooper*

---

"Unfortunately, after only one year, I realized the job was not going to work. My mental health challenges began to affect my work and I found it necessary to leave."
– Caroline –

---

I have lived with depression and anxiety for most of my life. I received treatment on and off over the years but nothing consistently, until I had postpartum depression after my third of four children was born. It was a scary time. I was afraid for myself and my kids. Getting help was not an option. I was on medication and went to therapy for about a year until the most severe symptoms subsided. But I still had many moments where I didn't feel "right." I knew I was a very emotional person, but I also lived in denial about the seriousness of my problems.

In 2002, shortly after turning 40, I entered an outpatient program in the trauma unit of a local psychiatric hospital. This was a result of an emotional breakdown attributed to post-traumatic stress disorder (PTSD) and a diagnosed mood disorder. Looking back, I can clearly see how God used this experience to bring healing into my life. It began with my journey of hope and recovery.

After this intensive treatment, I continued in therapy for several years. Journaling was an important part of the recovery process. Eventually, these writings were used as inspiration for my first book, In This Corner: Battling Depression from Inside the Ring. I wrote it for very selfish reasons; it is a reminder of my journey to victory. For many years now I have worked with a psychiatric nurse practitioner to manage my medication. I see a therapist as needed.

It is amazing how fast time flies. The years passed and my husband and I entered the empty nest stage. In the spring of 2016, about 14 years after my time in the psychiatric hospital, I learned about a certification program through the Missouri Department of Mental Health for 'mental health consumers': people receiving psychiatric treatment and living a recovery lifestyle.

This was a calling I could not resist. Within six months, I completed the training and passed the certification test to be a peer specialist. I did not hesitate to change careers, leaving a 10-year position in the marketing department of a large engineering firm.

As a peer with an employment services department, I supported the specialists who assisted clients with finding and maintaining employment. I also served as an advocate for the client from a peer perspective. Drawing from my personal experiences with mental health challenges, I encouraged clients to recognize there is hope for a fulfilling and productive life, even after being diagnosed with a mental illness.

It was a privilege and a blessing to work part time in the behavioral health field. Unfortunately, after only one year, I realized the job was not going to work. My mental health challenges began to affect my work and I found it necessary to leave. I am taking a break from working outside the home

As one of my first activities after leaving my job, I decided to do more research on mental health and find available resources. I went to the library to check out books on depression and bipolar. As I browsed the shelves, I became a little sad at the thought that this abundance of resources indicated that many people suffer from emotional trauma and mental illness.

Over the next few days as I began to read through the books, the Holy Spirit nudged me to consider some words that seemed to be repeated over and over. The same words that came to my mind to describe my life with mental illness: we 'suffer' from our condition. I suffer from bipolar II disorder. Even in the last paragraph I wrote that "many people suffer from mental illness."

I had never considered the significance of that little phrase before. Do I really feel like I'm suffering? No, I don't at this point of life. Does suffering have to be part of life, for anyone? Yes, we will have distress and extreme sorrow in life. We will grieve. We will be hurt, angry, lonely, and confused. But instead of dwelling on the pain, we can use those life experiences to make us stronger. It's not easy, but it is possible. I'm living proof of that truth.

I choose to believe that when we focus on the amazing grace and blessings we have in the Lord, we can live joyful, abundant lives! We will face challenges living with mental illness and it can be difficult It requires an extreme amount of work to overcome out-of-control emotions and learn to prepare for bad days. We may struggle with guilt over words or actions that might have hurt someone when we were in a 'mood.'

In addition to the trauma or illness we are dealing with, at one time or another, we will face tragedy, loss, illness, or other hardships that are part of life in this world. But none of these things have to elbow-out the promises of life in Christ. He has overcome the world and offers life without end, in His presence, in a place where there will be no more tears or suffering. We can persevere by relying on Him to be our source of strength.

> Jesus said, "Behold, an hour is coming, and has already come, for you to be scattered, each to chis own home, and to leave Me alone; and yet I am not alone, because the Father is with Me. These things I have spoken to you, so that in Me you may have peace. In the world you have tribulation, but take courage; I have overcome the world." (John 16:32-33, NASB)

From here forward, I'm going to be more careful in selecting words to describe how it feels to move through life with a diagnosed mood disorder. Mine is a joy-filled life! So what if I have bipolar? More importantly, I have the Lord Jesus Christ as my friend, my Savior, my God. When my eyes are focused on Him, how can I experience anything other than joy?

> I heard a loud shout from the throne saying, "Look, God's home is now among his people! He will live with them, and they will be his people. God himself will be with them. He will wipe every tear from their eyes, and there will be no more death or sorrow or crying or pain. All these things are gone forever." (Revelation 21:3-4, NLT)

In 2018, I formed a nonprofit, In God's Corner: Where Mental Health and Faith Connect, to continue the work God had invited me to perform. You can find out more information at www.ingodscorner.org.

# Loosing Daddy

## *by Jane Alexander*

I remember our mother saying on more than one occasion, "Don't we have a nice family?" These words were usually spoken during dinner time. My siblings and I did not know that there was an illness in our family: our father's illness and struggle with depression and alcohol addiction. Please understand that he was not a "mean drunk." I believe that his service during WWII (he was a bombardier) was a contributing factor to his suffering. I must emphasize that he was tormented mentally, physically and spiritually.

He travelled to an unknown place out of town a few times for "detoxification," and when we asked our mother about him, her reply was, "They are running tests. He will be home soon."

When I was 16, I knew there was something wrong with our father. He would come home from work in the middle of the day and take naps. He began to withdraw from the family. On January 27, 1974, I came home from school and could hear my brother sobbing. There he was at the top of the stairs, curled up in a heap. At age 14, he was the first person to know that our father's life had ended at age 49. Father left a note, "I'm sorry. I love you all."

My older sister was away at college in Vermillion, South Dakota. She was in the library when a chaplain approached her to tell her about our father.

Talking about suicide was a big taboo (this was the mid-'70s). I just remember I wanted everyone in the world to stop what they were doing and pay attention to me, if only for a few days. It is likely that our father suffered from bipolar disorder (manic depression, as it was called in the past) although there was no such diagnosis during that era.

I was diagnosed with bipolar disorder in 2007. I have learned to live with it and realize that it doesn't define me. Taking prescribed medications, keeping doctors' appointments and maintaining relationships are all important. I also have a strong church family.

Today there is a great deal of help for those who are struggling. Not only are there psychiatrists and psychologists, but there are therapists and support groups, such as NAMI (National Alliance for Mental Illness). Some churches are now offering anxiety and depression support groups. There is a National Suicide Prevention Lifeline, 1-800-273-TALK (8255), for those who are in a crisis.

I want to tell my story to encourage others. I want people to know there are mental health professionals, support groups, and many resources available across the nation. There is hope in this country for people to recover and be sustained in recovery.

> All praise to God, the Father of our Lord Jesus Christ. God is our merciful Father and the source of all comfort. He comforts us in all our troubles so that we can comfort others. When they are troubled, we will be able to give them the same comfort God has given us. (2 Corinthians 1:3-4, NLT)

Thank you for reading my essay. God bless you.

Jane Alexander

# I Am Not My Illness or My Trauma: I am a Child of God.

*by Susan M. Clabaugh*

---

"Recently, I decided to let my faith take over my brain. I am trusting the One who made me who I am. I choose to believe what God says about me instead of the world."
- *Susan* -

---

Mental illness and trauma have stigmas attached to them in our society; considered "bad labels" to people who do not understand. However, with the #metoo movement for recognition of women standing up to say, "Yes, I was sexually assaulted," things are starting to change for the world of sexual assault survivors. Survivors who have endured trauma and mental illness.

I am a sexual assault survivor. With the memories of my years of sexual abuse and assaults from childhood, came depression, anxiety, and post-traumatic stress disorder. I became unable to work due to my mental illness caused by my unprocessed childhood trauma. Trauma needs to be processed if we wish to get healthy.

Processing through trauma looks like seeing through a window into the past and talking and processing what happened with my Christian trauma therapist. He helps me process what happened as we work through each piece of each time abuse or rape happened. It's a step by step, slow process. If you take it too fast, your body will not process the trauma and will hold onto it. We use Dialectical Behavioral Therapy (DBT) skills to help keep me stable and able to function outside of therapy. Skills such as mindfulness, imagery, and emotional regulation, just to name a few. This helps keep me aware of what I am doing in the moment and not stay stuck in the past memories all of the time; helping with depression and anxiety as well.

I journal my thoughts and feelings each day, sometimes several times a day to help keep me "grounded" in the present day and to get my memories on paper so I don't ruminate on them. We work on my relationship with God in therapy too because it has been hard for me to comprehend God loves me and doesn't want perfection from me after so many years of abuse and rape. I also pray for God's help and guidance each day, and I know my therapist prays for me and himself too as we work in our sessions. God is leading our way.

Without properly working through my trauma as I've described I would not be able to move on with my life. The trauma would always be with me. It is so important to process ALL of it to become healthy.

It has been during my 10 years of my trauma work so far which I felt I was first labeled with my mental illnesses. Major Depressive Disorder (MDD), anxiety, and Post-Traumatic Stress Disorder (PTSD).

I let these labels define me, who I was, and what I did. I would introduce myself to medical professionals and people saying, "I have Major Depressive Disorder, anxiety, and PTSD because of severe childhood trauma. I lost my teaching career and had to go on disability because of it." I had it engrained in my brain this was who I was, and I couldn't do anything about it. I would always be this new "labeled" person.

Recently, I decided to let my faith take over my brain. I am trusting the One who made me who I am. I choose to believe what God says about me instead of the world. For now, I will still be on disability and need help. I have trauma work left to do. However, I am choosing to look at things differently.

After I work through my trauma, I might still have one of these conditions . I don't know. Even if I do, it will not label me. Only one thing defines me. I am a child of God.

---
So in Christ Jesus you are all children of
God through faith. (Galatians 3:26, NIV)

---

We are not MDD, anxiety, PTSD, codependent, bipolar, schizophrenic, or any other "label". There is no normal in life, but there is God. What defines us can only come from God. We are His children. We will never be our "trauma" or our "mental illness". We will always be children of God.

You can find and follow Susan online at:
Blog: http://susanmclabaugh.com
Twitter: @susanmclabaugh

---
"So in Christ Jesus you are all children of
God through faith." (Galatians 3:26, NIV)

---

Essays on Mental Illness

# A Comparison - Depression and a Man Lost at Sea

*A Poetic Reflection by Kaitlyn Wallace*

Waves.

Suffocating, terrifying, pitch-black waves that tear and rip and shred and crush every part of every piece of your soul. They suppress your hope, every reason to breathe is taken from you, breath by fading breath and there is nothing you can do about it but accept your fate and let the air be stripped from your lungs.

When the storm fades, you rise slowly to the surface, water-logged and gasping for your next breath, but alive. Always alive. The air is still. . . calm.

Sometimes storms are unpredictable, dragging you beneath the freezing waves in a matter of seconds. More often than not, you can't see the roiling clouds and flashing lightning until both are upon you, and suddenly,

you have no choice

but breath deep and hope you make it through another night.

# Prayer and Psychiatry

*by Zeta Combs Davidson*

---

"One by one, each of our closest friends and our pastor poured their hearts out to God on my behalf. More than one prayer was spiked with tears of compassion." – Zeta –

---

What got me through the dark hole of depression I found myself in? Time and again, I kept reminding myself that a medical professional had told one of my husband's close friends, Bill,

"Almost always depression is treatable if the right combination of medicines can be found."

I was beginning to wonder when I began my third combination of medications, and to make things even more laborious—one had to take each set for at least three weeks before a person could tell if they would 'kick in.' Days and nights came and went—never before had I missed being in front of my classroom more than a couple of days during my entire teaching career.

As prescribed, I attended an outpatient day psychiatric clinic while medicines were being tested on me. One day I was asked to journal—you will note the fragmented, sporadic thoughts that follow just as I recorded them:

It seems strange that I can't talk or think of anything to talk about. I wish I wasn't so withdrawn. I wish I wanted to eat. I wish very much for the medicine to work. This depression is so hard for me; I know it is so hard for my family and friends. Why can't I laugh or cry? It's not like I'm really sad, sad, but I'm certainly not happy. The personnel here at the hospital are nice to me but when I say anything, they say "Oh" or "Yes" and nothing really helps. It seems so unreal that all I can do is pray for help. I can't read my Bible with any understanding. Some people during group discussion use such foul language. I keep wondering why I'm being punished with this emotional zombiehood. I haven't done anything wrong. This first day at treatment is the strangest one of my life. When have I ever had a door lock behind me when I entered a building? When has my husband, Don, ever had to 'sign me in' anywhere? One girl, Ellen, remembered me from being a presenter in my classroom. She used to speak from Consumer Credit Counseling Services. The art project was so simple even a four-year-old could have done it. How can all this possibly help me? It has been a very long day and I did not know where or when to go between group times — others go outside to smoke or back to their rooms. I know a person is supposed to fight depression; I have no fight left in me. Patients here are so worried about when they'll get to smoke; how stupid that seems to me. The long walk was no exercise at all; I didn't even sweat . . .

During the final few days of my four weeks of 'day care,' still not sleeping, choking down only a few bites a day and not being able to make any decision—Bill's wife, Sandy, told my husband of their son's suggestion.

"Mom, we say we believe in prayer. Why don't you have a prayer meeting for Zeta?"

Don shared that prospects were dim for my attendance at any function, much less a prayer meeting in my behalf, but he agreed to the idea. To this day, I have no idea why I went. The probability is great that I attended out of courtesy to this longtime friend. Sandy sat just to my left in the group, and she started the meeting by reading a Scripture. Then, very tactfully, she said we would start praying around the group, beginning on her left and then she would conclude. This allowed everyone a chance to pray before the circle got to me. One by one, each of our closest friends and our pastor poured their hearts out to God on my behalf. More than one prayer was spiked with tears of compassion. Don was overwhelmed with gratitude for the love and support. I was still in a place where I could neither laugh nor cry, nor could I voice a prayer when it was my turn.

However, when I awoke the next morning, I was more like my "real" self than I had been in three months. The next appointment with the psychiatrist was early the next week. A still, small voice from deep within nudged me: *You are much better. You must share what I have done in your life.* When I met with the doctor, I credited the third combination of medications with working, but I also told of Sandy's prayer gathering for me on the previous Thursday evening. The doctor's reaction? A knowing smile and a big hug.

To this day, when asked about my struggle with depression—which I insist those I speak with treat it not as an illness to be 'swept under the rug of secrecy' but to be spoken about openly the same as any other illness—I credit both the combinations of medicines plus prayer for my deliverance of healing. Yes, it bothers me that my medical team insists that I take the medications for the rest of my life. I am more than glad to never to return to that awful black hole. Much more than ever before, I read this inspirational verse with confidence:

> The prayer of a righteous man is powerful and effective. (James 5:16)

# Perseverance: A Way of Life

*by Beth*

---

"Perseverance was never really a choice for me. Giving up was never an option."
– Beth –

---

I didn't realize my depression and social anxiety were such a problem until I experienced a series of traumatic events. Persevering through pain was a necessary part of my life.

I first recognized my depression in about 8th or 9th grade after an especially heart-breaking year. My grandmother died and my parents divorced around the same time. I was sad all the time and uninterested in activities of life. Although I confided in a friend, I did not initially seek medical help.

As an adult, I began to have problems at work in the education field. We had a student that was incorrectly placed and, because of it, suffered extreme behavior problems to the point of physical altercations. The other staff wanted to be oblivious and, when things finally got too bad to ignore, the student became a problem they dealt with by blaming me and isolating me continually.

In the beginning days of these problems I would drink more at night, always with dinner. That was my rationale. It could be 3-4 glasses of wine. I never considered myself having a problem with drinking, and I didn't want to go down that road and add to my other problems.

I decided it was time to talk to my mom. I began seeing a counselor off and on but was not really engrossed in the therapy. I went through a period where I ate very little and either filled myself with coffee to stop cravings or just went hungry.

My problems escalated to the point that I eventually left work and went on disability. After that, I became more regular with taking medicine and attending therapy sessions.

Part of perseverance is hope too. Hoping that if you keep pushing on enough that there is hope for better ahead.

I am on medication every day and am in therapy. Therapy sessions vary in times per month. In the beginning, it was once a week. Now I go from every two weeks to having 3-4 weeks between visits. The plan is working so far. It has been the better course of action than before. The medications are different from when I started and I have gone through many changes. But I like where I am now.

I have a great family that is loving and supportive. They wanted me around in their lives. No matter how horrible I may have felt, knowing they loved me made me push forward. My mom and her parents were really my rock, they were my everything (her parents have passed). They made me feel and let me know that I was their world. I didn't want to give that up.

Mom has been and always will be my best friend and biggest support. Before Papi (my mom's dad) died, mom met a guy she eventually married. He also fit into the family role of dad and demonstrated his love for me. My dad (stepdad) loves me like a daughter and openly calls me his daughter. My sister is older and we are best friends.

My dogs are my lifelines at home, too. Unconditional love from my family, and my dogs, help push me a lot harder, and want to be a better person.

# The Woman in the Mirror

*by Tess*

---

"I think the progress that has been made in understanding and treating mental illness since I was a teenager is remarkable, but we're still stumbling around in the dark."

- Tess -

---

When I was in high school, I remember my mom saying several times that she thought I was high because I was acting "giddy," and other times complained that I slept too much. A couple times I had some problem with my boyfriend and cried until it scared me because I couldn't stop, and I was sure I was crazy. Normal teenage stuff? Small town, 1970, mental health wasn't even a thing yet. So I learned not to cry.

Later, as an adult, I realized I'd had serious depression from the age of 17. Like many people, I have multiple mental health and addiction issues that I've learned to live with throughout my life: alcoholism (sober since 33 years old), ADD (attention deficit disorder), anxiety, social anxiety, eating disorder, PTSD (post-traumatic stress disorder), and DID (dissociative identity disorder). I was not formally diagnosed until my mid-30s, and then only with depression.

At 18, I had moved to Kansas City to be near my boyfriend. My oldest sister and I shared an apartment, and she introduced me to beer as a way to get to sleep. My relatives drank all the time, and my boyfriend loved clubs and music and booze. I was pretty much drunk or hung over for the next ten years.

I quit drinking when I found out I was pregnant with my first child and quickly got pregnant again while still nursing. After my second child was born, parenting and isolation overwhelmed me, and I started drinking again. When my oldest was two and I kept falling asleep on the couch with my two little kids in the house, I had to look in the mirror and call it: I was an alcoholic.

No one believed me. No one. Not even my dad who'd been in treatment twice by then and was sober again. Several friends told me it was probably a good idea to lay off, though, because they'd seen me start arguments and throw up in public. Even though I knew the truth, I couldn't go to AA by myself (social anxiety!) and no one would even drive me there and wait in the car. Now, of course, I recognize that most were hiding from their own addictions, and didn't want to be confronted with it. I am proud of the strength I found to fight that demon all on my own, constantly surrounded by temptation.

But, I still wasn't okay. I was doing my best to be a wife and mom but I'd never wanted those roles. I wanted the father's name on my kids' birth certificates so I took the vows and vowed to keep them. But without the true commitment, I soothed my misery with flirtations and relationships that walked just as close to that edge as possible without falling off the cliff. I kept this hidden from my counselors, until it got so involved that we came very close to divorce. But we didn't get any of the problems fixed, so that eventually happened anyway.

I realized how good I was at developing bad habits when I really tried to break off a serious relationship. I gained 15 pounds in two months. I realized I just kept trading one addiction for another. During this time I also went from my off-and-on cigarette smoking to a 3-4 pack per day habit, along with 10-15 cups of coffee a day. I was very good at developing very bad habits.

I had first tried counseling at about 31 because I was married, two kids, completely miserable. The first one I tried simply told me to be a better wife and mother, but my sister convinced me to see hers. I only went every month or two and I was always happier because I was talking to someone who was interested in my welfare. It took a couple of years for her to realize how serious my problems were. I didn't want meds but a couple of years later finally tried an antidepressant. It made me feel worse and my doc said nothing else would help either.

About seven years later, family deaths caused repressed memories of childhood sexual abuse to start surfacing and thoughts of suicide returned. I found a good counselor and new medication helped me cope for the next 18 months. Although it kept me out of the dark pit, my marriage ended.

---

*"I grew up with 'It's just the way he is,' and 'It's just the way I am,' and then I learned that's all a lie. We can all change, learn, adapt, and choose to do it in a healthy way."*

*- Tess -*

---

It wasn't long before I fell in love again. I got remarried and had two more kids. I had to stop my medication to nurse, but stayed fairly level even through some postpartum depression. My ex-husband withheld my kids from me but I survived.

My second husband and I both developed serious health issues, and he was diagnosed with mental disorders, but we survived. We were good partners, and went to God with the things we couldn't manage on our own, like raising teenagers. After 20 years, his leaving stunned me, but we are still friends.

I once had a counselor tell me she was crying for me, because I wasn't. I didn't know I was sad, or that my situation was sad. I thought I was just complaining. She told me she'd keep crying for me until I was able to do it for myself. That was 30 years ago and sometimes I still remember that and it helps.

The counselor who helped me the most said to let him know if I needed a hug. He was a big, burly bear and I knew he would be good at hugging. I ran into a patient in the waiting room that I knew from a survivors' group, and she'd told us her therapist just held her while she cried or threw tantrums. I never took him up on it, but if I saw him today I definitely would. I've come a long way.

> "Get encouragement and suggestions from people who seem to be at peace with themselves and their place in the world."
> –Tess -

My greatest challenge throughout my life was always feeling "behind." Behind everyone else who has achieved things, has good relationships, has learned what they need to function well, has energy to get things done, has the means and the fearlessness to go out and have fun or help other people. Behind the ones who can get off the couch, who don't take three naps and then still sleep eleven hours at night. Behind the people who learned the life skills at 30 that I just realized I even needed to learn at 60, or learned in kindergarten that I still don't have a clue about.

Now I am serious about taking care of myself: better food and less sugar, more sunlight, a little exercise. And PRAYER, PRAYER, PRAYER, PRAYER always, daily, many times a day. Sometimes I just don't have strength and I just need to stop whining. Sometimes I just don't have strength, and don't have the strength to work on regaining strength, and then I remember that God has strength enough for both of us, and He has stuff for me to do that I can't do from the floor.

> I pray that from God's glorious, unlimited resources he will empower you with inner strength through his Spirit. Then Christ will make his home in your hearts as you trust in him. Your roots will grow down into God's love and keep you strong. And may you have the power to understand, as all God's people should, how wide, how long, how high, and how deep his love is. May you experience the love of Christ, though it is too great to understand fully. Then you will be made complete with all the fullness of life and power that comes from God. Now all glory to God, who is able, through his mighty power at work within us, to accomplish infinitely more than we might ask or think. (Ephesians 3:16-21, NLT)

My advice to others living with addiction and mental health issues is simple. Stop holding on. Let go. Then look around and see what you really want for yourself. Pick up only the things that will help you get it, and get moving. Get encouragement and suggestions from people who seem to be at peace with themselves and their place in the world. Thank everyone who helps you along your way. Smile, even at yourself.

# Sleeping Free

*A Poem by Caroline S. Cooper*

My eyes reflect the moon's soft light
Shimmering darkness,
a restless night
  Helpless, shadowed dreams unfold
      Fantastic mysteries to be told
          To prisoners of the dream world's hold

Waking tears, a whispered prayer
God, I know
you're always there
  Let me rest beneath your wings
      Where your Spirit softly sings
          A quiet lullaby, and peace

Eyelids close, the moonlight fades
Welcome, darkness,
before the day
  His presence calms and comforts me
      His love, great love, how can it be?
          His grace assures me, I am free

Free to be me
Free to sleep

# Depression, Anxiety, Acceptance, Success
*by Sara*

---

"I like to compare how I experience depression to a gloomy haze that starts so subtly you can't detect it, and your eyes continue to adjust to the darkness creeping up around you, until all of a sudden you wake up and you can't function anymore and you realize you are totally surrounded by a dark cloud that has touched every aspect of your life." *- Sara -*

---

There are many of us who deal with mental health issues: anxiety, depression, bipolar, and many others. You are very far from alone. Recognizing it is truly one of the hardest parts.

My family has always been supportive and many extended family members deal with some form of mental illness. I am also fortunate to have a small group of close friends who were very understanding about what I was going through. I realize not everyone has this experience. I hope that any family members or friends reading this will recognize the importance of supporting their loved ones with mental illness.

I have depression and anxiety. I was diagnosed in my early 20s, only a few years ago. After my diagnosis, I had weekly counseling sessions for many months, then once a month for years. I eventually "graduated" to as-needed appointments. I am still taking my antidepressant, which has really helped me. I think the combination of therapy and medication has been incredibly effective. I have learned better coping skills and mindfulness, and actively employ these strategies to keep myself motivated. But getting to this point was not as easy as it may sound.

I believe it's important to share my story, but many times the stigma holds me back. There is an attitude of not wanting to seem weak and this makes me less likely to bring up my struggles. But to be fair, most people I've shared with have been very understanding. Perhaps some of what holds me back is my fear of how they will respond, as opposed to how people will actually respond.

Although I did not receive a formal diagnosis until a few years ago, I think the anxiety has been present in some form for most of my life. I have always had a tendency to be anxious. I am a chronic worrier and internalize a lot of my problems. This has been a part of who I am for as long as I can remember. I first became aware of my depression during my second year of law school.

> "Stress can be a good thing, and it's necessary in order to stimulate motivation. But I found myself with so much stress that my motivation tanked." - *Sara* -

A lot of things contributed to my stress. First, I had moved to attend law school. Being an hour away from home didn't seem too bad at first, but when I was used to living five minutes away, it really affected me to cut back my visits. Since my parents' divorce when I was a teenager, I had often felt responsible for caring for my immediate family, especially my mom. Not being able to check in as much as I would have liked made me feel extremely guilty and worried.

My siblings and I have always been very close, and being away from them also took its toll. Because of the difficult times we experienced, I had looked out for them maybe more than a typical older sibling would. I constantly worried about them, and whether they were doing okay without me (they were). On top of all of this, my grandfather had passed away, and I never fully allowed myself to grieve due to my busy schedule.

Law school is a competitive environment and it added to my stress. I was suddenly having to study every day as hard as I used to study the entire week of my college finals. School took over my life. But because of increasing anxiety and depression, I became unable to study. I just couldn't make myself do the things I needed to do. I couldn't even do the things I enjoyed. I started to avoid everyone in my life. It came to the point that I barely got out of bed, and was skipping class. When I did make myself study, I could only do it in front of the TV, using the distraction as a buffer. I failed a course. And then another one. When I was dismissed from law school, I finally admitted my need for help.

When my counselor gave me the diagnosis and asked if I was interested in trying medications, I started bawling. I finally released the pressure that had been building up for so long. I was upset, partly in denial, but also relieved because I knew these were steps that needed to be taken and would help me. I got started on an antidepressant and began Cognitive Behavioral Therapy (CBT, turning negative thoughts into positives); both were vital to my recovery.

Even with treatment, some days I just have bad days. It's something that is difficult to accept, especially when I feel that I am doing well overall. It's easy to just give up on those days and not fight to keep my motivation. The CBT and mindfulness skills (focusing attention on living in the moment) have been helpful in learning what factors affect my mood and how I can deal with stress more effectively. I started to time myself on tasks, especially studying, to make sure I wasn't letting myself drift along with no deadline.

After a few months of treatment, I appealed to the academics committee to reinstate me. I had to write a personal statement, get three letters of recommendation, and go in front of the committee to state why I felt I should be readmitted. I also had to be prepared to answer their questions. It was one of the most difficult things I have ever done. After voting, they reinstated me and I had to repeat my second year of law school. Since then I have not failed any courses, and thanks to my counselor and medication, I am enjoying the rest of my legal education and look forward to the future.

There are so many options now to try to better our situations, and the medical community continues to work to find more.


Sara used a website/app to help her stay focused:
- Habatica (formerly HabitRPG). It was very effective in keeping her daily schedule and getting things done. https://habitica.com

# Anxious Thoughts Turn to Hope
*by Cindy Richardson*

---

"Is it nature or nurture (or lack of) that produces anxiety in a child? Was my home so stressful that I picked up on it or is anxiety in the genetic make-up of my family? I don't know that I will ever have the answers to that question."
- Cindy -

---

I never wanted to be like my mom. I loved her dearly, but I saw her as my father's doormat. I imagined she cow-towed to him to avoid his explosive anger and the ensuing conflict. Looking back, I think I was an anxious kid from the start. I too, hated conflict, but there was much in my home growing up.

Is it nature or nurture (or lack of) that produces anxiety in a child? Was my home so stressful that I picked up on it or is anxiety in the genetic make-up of my family? I don't know that I will ever have the answers to that question. I do know that growing up I was painfully shy in a group and avoided being in front of any group for any reason. I also know that my grandmother took "spells" and "nerve pills" to prevent them. My mother followed in her steps and sadly I began down the same path.

As a child, the thought of being without my mom produced great anxiety. If anxiety didn't make me physically sick, I feigned illness whenever my mom couldn't come on a field trip, when I had to give a speech, or when life's demands got too much for me. I recall one evening when my parents got ready to go to dinner with friends for a rare evening out. I begged, cried, and even began to try to make myself sick in the bathroom to prevent her leaving. No wonder my digestive tract is a mess today.

Looking back, during childhood I took Pepto-Bismol at an alarming rate. The pink cocktail became my friend, my security, my go-to for moments of anxiety. I began to take it preventively, just in case I might have a stomachache. We should've bought stock.

Food is a snare to me. In my quest to overcome sugar addiction and get a handle on portion control I am realizing that I began turning to it for emotional comfort at a young age. I recognized this as one embarrassing memory surfaced.

For weeks I'd looked forward to spending the night at a close relative's house knowing I could take the pink bottle with me. She made everything seem special in my six-year-old world. This time, it was my favorite dessert; chocolate pudding served in cute little cups. I quickly enjoyed the first serving and asked for seconds. Hesitantly, she gave me another, then tried to talk me out of the third serving I began asking for. *"It wouldn't be good for you."* she said. *"It might even make you sick."* she warned.

I'll never know if it was out of a desire to please me, or perhaps to stop the whining and pouting I most likely displayed which caused her to give me a third serving. What I do know, is she was right. Eating 3/4 of a box of chocolate pudding *wasn't good* for me and *it did make me sick*; in the middle of the night, all over myself and the beautiful pink sheets in the princess pink bedroom, where I no longer felt like a princess. What causes a six year-old to be gluttonous? Did food feed an emotional emptiness?

While there are a lot of unanswered questions about my childhood anxieties, I started to get some answers when I became a Christian as an adult.

Life became overwhelming when I was a young mom. As a new believer, I knew nothing of spiritual attacks or how to fight spiritual warfare. My father died of cancer when I was 15. I feared I too would die of cancer. Every ache, pain, sickness and spasm created anxiety feeding into the narrative that I would develop cancer. My thoughts were unfounded and irrational, none the less very real to me. They began to consume my waking thoughts, and then rob me of a good night's sleep. Fear and anxiety caused stress leading to more physical ailments. When no medical basis could be found, it only fueled the fire of fearful anxiety.

The cycle began to take its toll on my well-being. With constant stomachaches and nausea, I consumed less and less food. Depression was creeping around the fringes of my anxiety and I felt weighed down, unable to do anything past automatic responses to routine actions. I lost interest in eating and consequently, lost 30 pounds. I lived in my pajamas without care. I had no joy and little faith to combat the fear threatening to reach in and steal my life.

By this time full blown panic attacks had set in and I felt like I was going crazy. I didn't know they were panic attacks, I thought I was dying. My wake-up call was when my husband thought I should check into a mental facility. The stigma was frightening to me. I remember my mother being confined to her bedroom for days on end. At one point I recall her absence, is that where she'd gone? Would that happen to me? Determined not to follow in her footsteps, I sought out my pastor.

Until then, pride kept me suffering in silence. Christians aren't supposed to be anxious, fearful, or depressed, are they?

I can remember meeting with the pastor as if it was yesterday. Trying to keep tears at bay, I started out my conversation with "I love my mother, but I never wanted to be anything like her, and here I am, exactly like her." His first response held the key to me overcoming anxiety, fear, and depression. "What you think and focus on, you often become."

My life seemed living proof of the truth found in Proverbs 23:7

> As a man thinketh in his heart, so is he.
> (Proverbs 23:7, KJV)

I had been so focused on the fearfully negative that I couldn't get out of the downward spiral. No wonder scripture tells us in Philippians 4:8 to think on things that are true, noble, right, pure, lovely, excellent, or praiseworthy. I began to realize that the more energy I used to focus on *not* becoming like my mother still centered my thoughts on her weakness thereby leading me down the same path she'd taken. Did she start with a similar journey of not wanting to be like *her* mother?

My pastor introduced me to Neil Anderson's book, *Victory Over Darkness*. It opened my eyes up to the spiritual forces of darkness lurking around, waiting for opportunities to kill, steal, and destroy believers. If Satan can influence our thoughts without our awareness we experience problems without the tools necessary to fight back. I once heard a speaker say, "Sow a thought, reap an action, sow an action, reap a habit, sow a habit, reap a life, sow a life, and reap a destiny."

I didn't want my destiny to included anxiety, panic attacks, or joyless living. And I didn't want to leave the same legacy to my children. I began to see a Biblical counselor who taught me how to renew my mind with God's word. Ephesians 6 gives us the blueprint to fight spiritual battles. She taught me to recognize signs of an attack so that I could defend myself against the enemy's schemes. Learning to be proactive in prayer, memorizing and meditating on scripture, and setting my thoughts on truth saved my mind and therefore my life.

---

Finally, be strong in the Lord and in the strength of His might. Put on the full armor of God, so that you will be able to stand firm against the schemes of the devil. For our struggle is not against flesh and blood, but against the rulers, against the powers, against the world forces of this darkness, against the spiritual forces of wickedness in the heavenly places.

Therefore, take up the full armor of God, so that you will be able to resist in the evil day, and having done everything, to stand firm. Stand firm therefore, having girded your loins with truth, and having put on the breastplate of righteousness and having shod your feet with the preparation of the gospel of peace; in addition to all, taking up the shield of faith with which you will be able to extinguish all the flaming arrows of the evil one. And take the helmet of salvation and the word of the Spirit, which is the word of God. (Ephesians 6:10-17, NASB)

---

I learned that praising God when I didn't feel like it was obedience, not hypocrisy. I learned that when my faith was weak, I could ask God to increase it. I began to know God more intimately and trust his faithfulness.

Then one year I embarked on a particularly hard season of life. My mother was diagnosed with Alzheimer's, my sixteen year-old daughter left our home to live with her boyfriend's family. We were ecstatic when she wanted to return home only to find out one month later she was pregnant. Unable to turn to my mom for comfort, I reached out to my oldest sister. As a cancer survivor, she'd learned to put life into perspective and while I hated my circumstances, she helped me see the bigger picture than just the current moments of disappointment and pain. Then she was killed in a car accident.

I was undone that year. I couldn't curtail the sadness. Tears were ever on the brim and some days they flowed so free that I could barely see. By God's grace I journaled my questions, frustrations and prayers and kept seeking answers in God's word. When my faith faltered, God began to whisper hope into my spirit. One morning in my journal he gave me this acronym for hope: Hang Onto Possible Endings.

There is a saying, "The bend in the road isn't the end of the road, unless you refuse to take the turn."

> HOPE = Hang on to Possible Endings.
>
> "Hope helped me take the turn and wait patiently for God to work all things for my good and his glory. Hope was the gateway to peace. When combined with faith, hope restored the joy of living."
>
> *- - Cindy - -*

You can find and follow Cindy online at:
www.cindyrichardson.org
https://www.facebook.com/authorcindyrichardson/
Instagram @crichardsonhope
https://www.facebook.com/groups/373594460088674/

# Grief and Tears
*Poems by Cindy Richardson*

## Grief's Obsession
Oh God,
The pain is intense.
I can't hold back the tears.
I can't enjoy the moment.
Grief is ever present,
Hovering over me.
Affecting every decision,
Underlying every reaction.
Please bring back the JOY.

## Tears
Tears fall.
Sometimes for no apparent reason at all.
Yet,
He knows.
He's seen it before.
He's got it covered.
He's got a plan.
I am in His hands.
Tears slow.

---

You've kept track of my every toss and
turn
through the sleepless nights,
Each tear entered in your ledger,
each ache written in your book.

(Psalm 56:8, MSG)

---

# Jane's Journey

*by Jane Alexander*

Twelve years ago, my life changed in a very frightening, unexpected way. As an x-ray technologist (a position I held for twenty years), you are required to lift, and transfer and push patients and x-ray equipment for most of the day. Being of Irish descent, I am six feet tall and would often have to stoop or use body mechanics that were not healthy for my spine. Simply put, I am not as close to the ground like so many others.

I began to experience pain in my lower back, and my doctor ordered some physical therapy. While it helped, I still had pain but wanted a conservative approach to treating my back. Next we tried acupuncture, then massage. I finally resorted to steroid injections, since I had heard some positive things.

The first injection didn't work. I went back a week later for the second injection and three days later I went into a steroid rage. My behavior was volatile and very unpredictable. All of this occurred while I was on the job.

Human Resources became involved and I found myself sitting across from the HR director her office.

"Jane, we'd like you to get some help."

She subtly and slowly pushed a consent form across her desk hoping I would agree to medical treatment. After refusing to sign the form, I was told to go home. Instead I went to the hospital gift shop and spent $75 on items I didn't even need.

I went back to my department and it was obvious to my coworkers that I was out of control and irrational. My husband and daughter came to the hospital and they urged me to go to the ER. Again, I refused to get help.

One of the employees finally persuaded me to go and pushed me in the wheelchair to the ER.

My behavior was no better in there and actually worsened. I remained aloof, as if nothing bothered me. And then I snapped and wanted to go home. I wanted to go home.

In the meantime, the psychosis manifested itself. Looking back, I don't believe it could have been any worse. I became psychotic and thought my family and the hospital staff were playing tricks on me. And I still had to wait for more intensive help. I stayed in the ER because there were no empty beds in nearby psychiatric hospitals. Finally, I was taken to a hospital in Kansas, an hour away from home, with my family following the ambulance. It was 9:30-10:00 pm. I was thinking ,"Where am I? Where am I."

The next morning I woke up in my work clothes, and still didn't know where I'd been taken. I started reciting the 23rd Psalm.

> The LORD is my shepherd; I shall not want. He makes me to lie down in green pastures; He leads me beside the still waters. He restores my soul; He leads me in the paths of righteousness. For His name's sake. Yea, though I walk through the valley of the shadow of death, I will fear no evil; For You are with me; Your rod and Your staff, they comfort me. You prepare a table before me in the presence of my enemies; You anoint my head with oil; My cup runs over. Surely goodness and mercy shall follow me All the days of my life; And I will dwell in the house of the LORD Forever. (Psalm 23, NKJV)

That evening, my family gathered around me as if waiting for me to go to sleep. Maybe they did not want me to fall asleep alone. In my mind, I believed my pastor was also present. He was a comforting presence and was waiting for other patients to sleep so he could pray with me. In reality, he wasn't there. I wondered,

"Could this be an angel watching over me?"

In the hospital, patients waited their turns to visit the psychiatrist. There were few activities to keep me from being bored.

When I was released, I continued to have issues. I was working with a psychiatrist who tried adjusting my medication. I was still having manic episodes, but because I wanted to feel normal, I went back to work. But, I experienced episodes of rage and continued having manic episodes. But I continued working until October. As a result of my behavior, on October 12, I was finally escorted out of the building.

The ups and downs continued for over six months, April to October 2007. Finally, in October I found a psychiatrist. My first words were, "Please, please help me." He was calm and gentle and I began to feel less anxious about the appointment. I told him, "There's something wrong with my mind." For the first time, I was given a diagnosis of bipolar disorder.

The last week of October, I entered a partial hospitalization as recommended by my doctor.

It probably took a couple of years before I felt stable and settled into a new routine. With the right medicine and a kind and effective doctor, real healing began.

One recommendation I have when first noticing mental health issues is to visit a pastor. Consult with him. Let him pray for you. Have him recommend a therapist or other means of help. Remember that God is with you through every experience in life, even on a journey from a dark pit and back to the mountaintop.

It's been 12 years and the events are still vivid. I thank God I'm in a place of stability. My family is supportive and understanding. As the mental health coordinator for In God's Corner Ministry, I have a sense of purpose.

---

> Be anxious for nothing, but in everything by prayer and supplication, with thanksgiving, let your requests be made known to God; and the peace of God, which surpasses all understanding, will guard your hearts and minds through Christ Jesus. (Philippians 4:7, NKJV)

# "Keep Your Powder Dry"
## *by Bill*

---

> "Depression. Suppressed anger. Attention deficit hyperactivity disorder (ADHD). I lived with those conditions for many years before receiving a diagnosis."
> - *Bill* -

---

In 1989, I lost my job. Not the first or last time that happened. That same year, I went to the ER because of high blood pressure. With the stress in my life, I wasn't surprised that my blood pressure had spiked. I was surprised when the doctors told me the blood pressure problem could be caused by depression. I wish I'd been able to share the news with someone, but I felt as if I had no one to confide in. I would have to do my best to handle this on my own.

Over 10 years later, I was diagnosed with ADHD. This was a scary time because I could not contain my anger and my wife and children bore the brunt of it. I am still ashamed of it and I fight it every day. I don't always win the fight.

We don't always understand why certain things happen. But I know my anger issues stem from a childhood full of mental and emotional abuse, by both parents. In fact, I believe the trauma of being treated in such a way was the underlying reason I had struggled with mood swings and rage throughout my life. Even now, many years later, I am still affected by the way I was treated by my parents.

Mom knew I was a dreamer and I had big plans.

Whenever Dad heard me discussing my dreams, his response would always start with something like "let me tell you what's wrong with that idea" or "let me tell you why that won't work."

My mother passed away five years ago. I sat beside her hospital bed when she died, but in the five years since, I've yet to shed the first tear. She always used guilt to manipulate me. When we were little kids, she always treated my siblings and I like we were in the way. Later on in our lives, she was good about everyone being treated equally. Every child who attended a birthday party would get something. This included our friends.

I interact with my father almost every day. He still verbally abuses me in an attempt to hurt my mother, even though she is gone. I have to be careful not to let him "push my buttons."

Even now, Dad does not treat my children equally, because he knows I adore them. On birthdays and some holidays, he'll give money to his favorite niece and to one of my children, but not the other two. Right in front of them!

I have only been seeing my psychologist for about three years and that has been a big help! My faith in God has kept me strong and so has the patience of my family. I feel my treatment plan combining medication with therapy is 99% effective.

I still have anger issues at times, but I have to deal with them. My greatest challenge is to not let my mental illness affect my immediate family. It's hard because the natural inclination is to let my guard down around them. I should be able to be myself with them without causing them pain, but it's not always that easy.

The best advice I can offer to others is to, "Trust God but keep your powder dry." In other words, God provides for our needs, but we still need to be ready to fight with an effective weapon.

## Editor's Note

I was inspired by the quote this gentleman used as his advice to others, "Trust God but keep your powder dry." Since I was not familiar with it, I did some research to better understand its meaning. Here's what I found.

---

"Trust God and keep your powder dry" is a saying that dates back to the English Civil War and is attributed to Oliver Cromwell. It is a statement that would remind us that faith in God does not make one irrational or irresponsible. Trusting God does not relieve the soldier of the duty to have a fully functioning firearm. Trusting God for protection does not rule out the use of means or responsible human behavior. It must be remembered that looking to God does not equate to blind trust or to a kind of fatalism that excuses us from thinking hard, acting wisely, or going to others for help or counsel." – *Pastor Philip DeCourcy -- https://www.ktt.org/resources/truth-matters/ keep-your-powder-dry*

---

The Bible has many stories of God's people putting faith in God first as well as taking responsibility for developing the necessary disciplines for living a Christian life. The book of Nehemiah contains one of those examples.

*Nehemiah*

The setting of this story is Jerusalem when the Israelites were allowed to return after 70 years in captivity. A group of men, led by Ezra and Nehemiah, worked to rebuild the wall around Jerusalem, which had been broken and burned by Israel's enemies. But not everyone was happy the wall was being repaired.

---

When our enemies heard that we were aware of their plot and that God had frustrated it, we all returned to the wall, each to his own work. From that day on, half of my men did the work, while the other half were equipped with spears, shields, bows and armor. The officers posted themselves behind all the people of Judah who were building the wall. Those who carried materials did their work with one hand and held a weapon in the other, and each of the builders wore his sword at his side as he worked. But the man who sounded the trumpet stayed with me. Then I said to the nobles, the officials and the rest of the people, "The work is extensive and spread out, and we are widely separated from each other along the wall. Wherever you hear the sound of the trumpet, join us there. Our God will fight for us!" (Nehemiah 4:15-20, NLT)

---

God would fight for His people, Israel, but they needed to be prepared as well.

This is exactly what we have to do when coping with our mental health conditions. God gives us the strength and power we need to face hardship, and we also need to use the resources and tools available to us as we take responsibility for our mental health.

"Trust in God, but keep the powder dry."

In other words, trust in God, but be prepared for the battle.

# Hopeless and Hopeful
*Poems by Cindy Richardson*

## Hopeless
Lord,
My heart breaks,
My soul awakes,
To the dread,
She's gone.
How did it happen?
Slowly over time?
Or was it always there and
I never took the time
To see it?
This rebellious heart,
Focused on self,
Bent on her way.
And coming back?
No way,
She's gone.

## Hope Says
Sad…
    Mad….
Will I ever get glad?
Hope says, someday.

## Hope Changes Everything
Grief.
Lost innocence,
    broken dreams,
        unknown future,
            tainted past.

Jesus.
Redemption found,
    new dreams,
        bright future,
            forgiveness.

Hope.

Essays on Mental Illness

# Cyclothymia
*by Judith Vander Wege*

---

"Although the highs and lows of cyclothymia are less extreme than those of bipolar disorder, it's critical to seek help managing these symptoms because they can interfere with your ability to function and increase your risk of bipolar I or II disorder." - *MayoClinic.org* -

---

Cyclothymia—or cyclothymic disorder—is a rare mood disorder, similar to bipolar but not as extreme. In cyclothymia, moods alternate between periods of depression and hypomania, an elevated mood. Cyclothymia can straddle the line between mental illness and normal variations in mood and personality. Some people with mild symptoms are highly successful in life, driven by their hypomania to express individual talents. On the other hand, chronic depression and irritability can ruin personal and professional relationships.

I think I've had cyclothymia all my life, but I didn't receive diagnosis and treatment until after age 65. Perhaps I could have avoided a lot of heartache in my relationships if I'd had treatment earlier. After a divorce in 1981, my life was a mess for several years. I used to think the depression I felt resulted from the emotionally painful situations in my life, and from chronic health issues. Later, when my health and circumstances improved and there seemed no outward reason for the depression, I sought medical help to explain it.

For a couple of years, I'd had a therapist who helped by letting me talk out my feelings. We didn't know I had cyclothymia, but it helped to know she cared and would pray for me. She helped me figure out how to act in some challenging relationships.

In 1994, I'd found out I had mercury toxicity. The doctor, an expert in chronic diseases, prescribed many supplements to help get the mercury out of my system. At his recommendation, my dental fillings were replaced with composite fillings in 1995. (Dentists usually use amalgam fillings, which are made up of mercury, silver, and other metals. The composite fillings, which are white, don't have any mercury.) He also prescribed a small dose of lithium, saying my hair analysis showed a lithium deficiency. My health gradually improved under his care over the next eleven years. Meanwhile, I had another heartache in 2003 when my husband died of cancer.

In 2006, I remarried and moved to Iowa. It was a good situation and my physical health improved while the mercury (which has a 15-year half-life) was eliminated. Therefore, I wondered in the following years why I still felt depressed. My lithium prescription had run out, so I went without, then noticed my symptoms got worse. Finally, my doctor sent me to a psychiatrist to get an accurate diagnosis. The psychiatrist said I had cyclothymia and prescribed a larger dose of lithium. I began to feel "normal." Now that I have the proper dose of medication, I feel that I am an emotionally healthier, more out-going, and less paranoid person.

> "Get medical help, psychiatric help, spiritual help, whenever you suspect something is wrong. We aren't expected to muddle through life without help." – *Judith* –

As a Christian, my faith has made an incredible difference in my recovery. God, in His wisdom and mercy, worked through my depression, heartaches, and mistakes to teach me how to draw closer to Him, to depend on Him. He gave me the ability to write poems and songs which brought me joy. He taught me through His Word and prayer to trust Him wholeheartedly, then led me to solutions and continues to guide and uphold me.

## Editor's Note

Judith Vander Wege is an accomplished writer and a member of the same writer's group I attend: Heart of America Christian Writers Network (HACWN) in the Kansas City area. She has graciously shared with us one of her poems of hope and healing.

# Healing Elements
*A Poem by Judith Vander Wege*

A soft, gentle breeze caresses my skin,

Uplifting my spirits, it soothes me within.

I gaze at the sunset, with awe contemplate

the marvelous beauty my God did create.

Music is healing, music gives wings

To soar above problems this troubled earth brings.

Lord, You sent the music, You give the sunsets,

You are the breeze to my soul.


You can find and follow Judy online:
- http://judithvanderwege.com
- http://judithvanderwege.com/blog
- http://Facebook.com/judithvanderwege


Judy recommends the following books. They can be found on Amazon.
- Healing Damaged Emotions by David Seamands
- Something More by Catherine Marshall

# Hope for Depression Healing
## *Zeta Combs Davidson*

---

"I read my own medical records as if I were standing over to the side seeing descriptors of someone else." – Zeta –

---

What can create more pain for a person than a broken ankle requiring a plate and seven screws to patch? When I had that broken ankle, the pain was intense, but surgery and medication brought relief. For me the emotional pain of a depression breakdown was constant and, at the time, seemed to be unending.

I knew exactly what was happening—my speech was slowed; my physical movements were slowed. I could neither eat nor sleep—at the deepest point, I went four days and nights without sleeping. A bite of a peanut butter sandwich stuck in my throat like a mass of glue that would not go down. For two months, I still got up every morning, showered, put on makeup, did my hair and made my way to the high school classroom where I'd never missed a day for illness before. Then one day, I woke my husband, Don, and said, "I can go no farther." He called my school and searched for our primary care doctor's phone number. Bless his heart, Dr. Terry Calhoun knew what I looked and acted like when I was healthy. He prescribed some medicine and referred me to a psychiatrist. You guessed it. I had to wait three weeks to have the appointment. Those twenty-one days dragged on, one into another. I wasn't sleeping, but I hardly left my bedroom.

My weight plummeted to 106 lbs. My dear daughter-in-law found some cute size 6 tan chinos at a local thrift store and brought them by. My reaction? "What will I wear these with?" (Talk about distorted thinking.)

Her reaction? "Zeta, tan chinos will go with almost every top in your closet." She probably thought, "And there's not tons of extra fabric hanging off your behind."

My daughter came home from college and no Christmas decorations were in our house—always by the day after Thanksgiving, every room was decorated to honor the birthday of Christ. She unpacked the tree, ornaments, placed the collection of nativity scenes about the rooms. I hardly noticed. My adult son and a close friend were called to stay with me when Don had to be gone—fortunate now that I think about it, he owned his own business and could set his own hours.

The day finally came. My husband, Don, took me to see Angela Olomon, MD. Her immediate reaction? "Why did you not tell my receptionist this was an emergency?" At some point, I never knew when, she advised my husband to lock and secure all medications at our house, even the Tylenol. Her diagnosis' plan was to start me on two new different depression meds, arrange for me to see the psychologist in her office and for me to attend a month-long out-patient mental health clinic. Long story short, three long, at least to me, months later and three different kinds of depression prescriptions, my emotional pain improved.

Depression medications, for the most part, take time to take effect. Each set had to be taken for at least three weeks before evidence might be seen of depression lifting. I read my own medical records as if I were standing over to the side seeing descriptors of someone else.

Our closest friends gathered for pleading prayer. To this day, I know, without a doubt—the combination of the correct medications and prayer were my lifesaver. I've asked my new primary care physician if newer depression meds that had fewer side effects would work for me. His response? "The combination of these two drugs work for you; I would not be about to change them."

What has happened as a result of sharing this mental health situation and these facts? Depression affects so many at times in life. Time after time, friends come to ask,

"Zeta, will you please talk with my sister, my uncle, my son. . ."

No, I don't share every ugly detail, but I listen to how each are feeling and share what part of my story seems right for the time. For most, I always include, "I will never stop taking my medication (I was advised never to.) and I found great help by doing the exercises in the revised edition of David D. Burns, M. D., <u>Feeling Good—New Mood Therapy</u> which uses cognitive behavioral therapy in ten categories. In a nutshell, a person records his/her distorted thoughts on the left side of a sheet of paper and then writes down on the right a rebuttal sentence that shows what correct positive thoughts and reality really are.

I also ask, "Are you getting any physical exercise?" You can guess the most often reply. Twenty minutes of walking or other exercise each day replaces endorphins in the brain that have been completely used up during the time frame of 'fighting' depression.

Finally, I share the verse that I originally shared at a thank you session of close friends who had gathered for prayer on my behalf.

> "The prayer of a righteous person is powerful and effective" (James 5:16b NIV).

Yes, observing my own ankle with the foot dangling off to the side was excruciating. But if you've been there, you will agree—nothing matches the deep emotional pain of untreated depression. There is hope—an ankle can be fixed. And a brain and its emotions can be fixed—using vigilance, individualized medication and prayer.

# From Prison to Purpose
## by Joshua Callahan

> I stopped letting my circumstance dictate my emotions and started learning the importance of thankfulness in all situations like the apostle Paul talks about so much.
> - *Joshua* -

I grew up going to a Christian school in Chattanooga TN. Most of my life I was pretending to be a Christian but not living like one. As an adult, I served in the army for a 15 month deployment to Iraq. Like many soldiers, that experience caused trauma in my life.

In 2016, my wife and I were going through a divorce. She falsely accused me of some bad stuff to gain custody of our 5 children. I was miserable and blamed God for my failed marriage. Because of her claims I spent 23 months in jail on a no bond awaiting trial. About a month before jail I cried out to God one last time asking Him to intervene and change me. I did not get an answer. I eventually gave up on God and church.

That first month in jail was honestly horrible. I wanted to die but finally realized I could not live my life hating my ex-wife and continuing to sit in pity. I was looking at life without parole if found guilty and decided to serve God no matter what happened with my circumstances. I decided to forgive my ex-wife and pray for her and my children. I decided to use my time wisely and started daily bible studies. I stopped letting my circumstance dictate my emotions and started learning the importance of thankfulness in all situations like the apostle Paul talks about so much.

I became more involved with other inmates and their families. I started counseling them and praying with them, and also had opportunities to preach.

Although jail wasn't what I would have ever asked for, here I found what I needed. Before jail I was selfish and cared about myself and money more than anything else. God saved my life through this experience in jail, and for that I am thankful.

Before trial date arrived, God finally answered my prayer. The district attorney thought something wasn't right and decided to do some more digging. He concluded I was innocent and dismissed my case. He also expunged my record.

I still have not seen my 5 kids in a few years but I am fighting to see them and hopefully soon we will be back together again.

Because of my interest in prisoners, I served as the chaplain for the national veterans association for the state of Kansas. I would like to someday minister at the local jails and hope to still be able to help inmates.

# Surviving Home With my Mother

*Stories and Poems by Rosie Maureen*

---

"I finished school at 17 because I skipped a grade. A few weeks before I graduated I went down to the salvation army and prayed for my soul." -Rosie Maureen-

---

I had a rough start in life. From my youngest years I was exposed to some of the worst in human nature. My mom enjoyed a stable marriage but when my dad passed, Mom lost her own way, delving into drugs, prostitution and violence.

I seemed to be equipped to handle this because God saw me through even though my growing up years were never easy. God directed and enabled me to rise to every occasion.

One summer, my mother went "AWOL," leaving me with only one kind of meal, Vienna sausages. Today, I still strongly dislike them, not even able to look at them.

One day, while being playful as a young child, Mother became inexplicitly enraged, kicking me down the stairs.

Thankfully, I survived but the pain of that memory still hurts. I began getting shuffled about the Foster Home Care System. I was impossible to "tame" and easily managed to go "missing." I was tied into that system until I reached 18 years of age.

To this day, I devote my time to causes that directly benefit the extremely disadvantaged including feeding and clothing the homeless in a nearby encampment. I never miss a major holiday, including Easter, Christmas and Thanksgiving Day. I'll be there, helping to serve food, beverages, including coffee, sodas and the like. There are over 700 people in this location.

I believe in protesting and advocating for things that help others with no voice, including many homeless veterans.

I also dedicate at least one day per week in gathering flowers. I bring them home, weed out the bad, and transform the displays. I then take them to folks in area senior centers, and into private homes, sending cheer into lives that otherwise have little to none.

Some are dying, afflicted with cancer and other diseases or disabilities. I take this God-given responsibility seriously and try not to skip a beat, especially towards all who really need a cheerful smile and a gentle flower.

During all of this, I raised two children and cherish every opportunity to still be their friend and confidant.

And all while battling the onslaught of Sarcoidosis. [Author's note: Sarcoidosis is an inflammatory disease that affects multiple organs in the body, but mostly the lungs and lymph glands.] But, I'm a private type, not usually indulging my private battles in conversation. Please pray and support me as I continually seek to Honor - with my very life - my Lord and King, Jesus Christ.

## A story and poems about Mom

My mother never said she loved me
She could never say she loved me
because the booze got in the way
preparing to be drunk, drinking and then recovering
from the drinks in order to do it again
took almost all of her time

> I adapted the way children do relishing the precious
> interludes of norm beneath the surface of the bitter.
> I would store each of her rare smiles in my memory like
> sweet apples in a dusty cellar - hoarded, as if against a
> coming famine because I loved her even if I never said it.

In re-reading this poem, it sounds like I was raised by a monster. I loved her, but love isn't blind so real love can hurt, even though it shouldn't.

We were all happy once. I am sure of it. I've seen the pictures. Man. Woman. Child.

When life became filled with sorrow, I would watch children play and wondered how that would feel to laugh and be free. I didn't let myself linger on the bad memories too long. I was just glad that I was alive.

My mother was an only child who came to the United States from Jamaica with her mother. She never really knew her mother because she died a few years after the move. My mother was placed in a group home. Tauntingly beautiful, exotic and alone, she was raped often by the man in charge of the home.

Therefore, by the time she ran away at 14, drugs were her cure for all that bothered her.

Five years later she met my father. Raised in a boy's home he was lonely for roots and a family as well. After a quick courtship, he took her for his bride, reformed her, and created me.

Then he died and life ended even as it went on. My

mother returned to drugs, it was what she knew. Soon she slipped into prostitution and sold drugs.

There were weeks when everything was peaceful. Those were the scariest times of all because I knew it couldn't last. She was manic, cooking birthday cakes when it wasn't my birthday, painting the walls bright yellow and then stopping and crying about the color. She would try to stop the booze. and then crack cocaine came around. Things became so bad that I could not believe it was real.

Sometimes the state took me away, but she would cry, take me back, and then have us move, six or seven times a year. She would beat men, they would beat her. I would try to stop it and then they would both beat me.

I loved her wildly, and would try to save her, dragging her out of bars, reminding her to take her birth control pills, wiping up the vomit. She would OD and I would try to hide all the drugs before I called the police. When I grew breasts she put locks on my bedroom door and told me if anyone broke in and tried to rape me, I should jump out the window. The idea of not having men in the house never occurred to her.

We moved for the 17th time. She opened a whore house taking in runaways and tricking them out as prostitutes. Sooner or later someone would call, close her down, and take me away just to give me back.

## Surviving Home With my Mother

My mother decided to settle down and marry again. It didn't work out so she divorced and tried four more times, six marriages in all.

> I would return as my mother
> Gently nurturing me
> from the first moment
> I would sing myself a lullaby, sweetly.
> Picking me up before I fell -
> whispering, "there, there."
> I would love me.

Junkies don't need to eat much so I rarely had real food. I used to climb out my window and search through the neighbor's trash for food scraps. Then something snapped and she decided the best thing to do was to die.

I would come home from school and see the bleeding wrists or the half empty bottle and save her.

After she ended up in jail, I was placed in foster-care. I finished school at 17 because I skipped a grade. A few weeks before I graduated I went down to the Salvation Army and prayed for my soul.

When my mother was released from jail, I told her of my dreams: college, and getting her real help. She refused and that was the last day I saw her. I hitchhiked to another state, got three jobs and sent her half the money. A few months shy of her 41st birthday she finally OD'd. She had just found out that her liver was failing. I was 21 and for the first time in my life I slept through the night. I have yet to shed one tear.

I loved my mother. Even after the cuts, broken bones, burns, that came with that costly love.

She made me call her by her first name, so she wouldn't feel old. That makes me saddest of all—I have never had the chance to call anyone Mother.

(WARNING: Heroin is one of the most addictive substances known to man. Only after repeated exposure to it, after it changes your physiology, will you feel the intense euphoria that junkies are obsessed with. By that time you will be so addicted that quitting will probably require professional treatment.)

---

### Always awake and dreaming of sleep
*to my mother*

To my mother I was born old and you so very young.
Not quite sure where you ended and I began
I was never sure if I could do anything right.
I spent the first half of my life getting very little sleep.

It was my duty to take care of you, I tried even while I did a less than perfect job. I never knew how not to navigate through whatever mood you wore at the time. Who you were that day meant who did I need to be for you. If I slept too long or too deep you might die and then what would I be?

Songless bird in a dirty cage flapping bloody wings so small I could never open the door. When you were not high you would cry for me to let you die - Such a heavy load to give a child. When you were drunk you would dance naked in the rain.
How could I have stopped you?

You were laughing, should I let you ?

The times you would stop breathing, needle in arm, I would hold my own breath until your heart began to beat. "Let her be awake in the morning and I'll be good" was my nightly prayer. I would whisper it until my eyes closed. Lord, I was so very tired. I can't remember all the names and places and faces and towns of my childhood.

I just remember you, smelling of cheap booze and men,
getting ready to dance topless in that club.
You would pull out the picture of us all and remind me
that you loved me once. "Never trust anyone, not even me."
You would laugh, your voice rolling like thunder
with your soft Jamaican accent.

Good night, at last tonight I will sleep.

# Hold Me Jesus
*Poems by Cindy Richardson*

## No Answers

Rolling tears, gently falling
Mirroring her choices.
How did we get here?
What lies does she believe as truth?
Will she ever see truth as Christ?
Will she find her way back home?
Will she choose to follow The Way back?
Hold me Jesus.


## Hope Believes

Words, words, words.
They can't express the depth of my sorrow.
Why is this sadness so overwhelming?
Where is my faith?
Where is my hope?
Lord, I don't see you working.
I want to have hope.
So, I call to mind your unfailing love, mercy, and grace.
Shower me with grace so it flows in me and through me.

Romans 4:18 "Abraham in hope believed."

Essays on Mental Illness

# Who Am I?

*by Caroline S. Cooper*

---

"Understanding my condition and getting the help I need have been crucial to accepting this part of my life." - *Caroline* -

---

I am a wife, mom, and grandma. I'm a writer and musician. I am a Certified Missouri Peer Specialist (CMPS). I am many things. But, I am not my diagnosis of bipolar disorder II. I am more than a mental illness. I am me! I live a full, productive, and blessed life. And so can you.

About a year ago, I created a mission statement to guide my personal life.

"To offer encouragement for life in a complicated world."

I want to support others the way I am supported. Family and friends love me unconditionally, with patience and compassion. I trust them to be available for me in a time of crisis. But not everyone has this kind of support. Many people need encouragement. If we listen to and observe the people in our lives, we may discover someone who needs to know we care. We can assure others they are more than their diagnosis, whatever that may be.

One of the many challenges we face every day is living a healthy lifestyle. Eating on the go, working too many hours, staying up late, and other factors affect our physical health and ability to cope with life's surprises. I know this from experience! The good news is, in these cases we can make changes, as difficult as they may be. We can get back on the healthy track.

Unfortunately, we don't always have control over our bodies and minds. Sometimes an unexpected diagnosis takes our breath away. For me, it is bipolar II disorder. After years of fluctuating between depression and anxiety, I was given the all-purpose diagnosis of a 'mood disorder.' It has only been within the past few years that I have been more accurately diagnosed with bipolar. Understanding my condition and getting the help I need have been crucial to accepting this part of my life.

Taking responsibility for our health and well-being is extremely important. We have to recognize there is hope for a better life and then take steps toward a more promising future by educating ourselves on our conditions. Along the way, we need to identify people who can give us support, even if that means stepping out of our comfort zone to find them. It may take some time, but once we can say, "I am more than a mental illness," or more than cancer, or fibromyalgia, or any other diagnosis, we can show the world who we really are.

---

You made all the delicate, inner parts of my body and knit me together in my mother's womb. Thank you for making me so wonderfully complex! Your workmanship is marvelous— how well I know it.
(Psalm 139:13-14, NLT)

---

# Appendix I – Be an Encourager

Originally published as a blog by Caroline S. Cooper, February 22, 2017

One of the biggest challenges for people who live with mental illness, or disabilities of any kind, is finding the support they need. Why? If we don't have firsthand experience, it can be difficult to understand what it is like to persevere through the daily challenges. That's just the way it is. How do we work through questions, concerns, and fears to effectively encourage loved ones with mental illness? The easy answer is, focus on the person and not the illness.

---

> "Society's perception is that the 'mentally ill' can't work, don't have healthy relationships, are to be feared, are not worthy of respect, and are relegated to the margins of society because they are 'different.' Yet they usually work tirelessly to regain a sense of self and a sense of peace."
> Dr. Nancy Dr. Nancy Kehoe, Wrestling with Our Inner Angels: Faith, Mental Illness and the Journey to Wholeness © 2009

---

Here are some practical tips to encourage hurting people. These suggestions are based on what I needed and experienced when I had severe depression. I will always be grateful for family and friends who reminded me I was loved.

1. *Communicate without judgment.*

As much progress has been made to reduce the stigma of mental illness, there still exists the belief that someone with depression should just "get over it." A person with an anxiety disorder may be told to "stop worrying all the time." Expressing unconditional love without judgment is essential.

2. *Be available.*

Even if you don't live nearby, you can show someone they are loved. A simple phone call or email might be just what he/she needs. Encourage them by simply being present.

3. *Spend time together.*

Don't wait for your friend to call you. They probably won't. Arrange a get-together, but do not stop by their home unannounced. A mom with postpartum depression may appreciate your offer to watch the kids while she takes a hot bath. Invite someone trying to hold on to employment to lunch. Enjoy each other's company to build a relationship of trust.

4. *Offer occasional household help.*

Occasional help with everyday responsibilities can motivate an individual to persevere. It is encouraging to know you have friends who care.

5. *Encourage participation in life.*

Isolation is a problem for many people. To draw this person out of isolation – share a meal, go for walks, take the kids on field trips, have a mom's chick-flick night or dad's bowling event. Show your friend that life is filled with blessings.

6. *Be honest about how you feel.*

Give your friend plenty of opportunities to talk, share, cry, and express feelings. Then, when it's your turn, tell the truth about how you feel. Are you worried? Scared? Mad? Frustrated? Don't share your feelings to cause a guilt trip, but to remind a friend you need encouragement, too. This can help a friend recognize the needs of others.

There is a secret weapon you can use on behalf of your friends, even if they don't realize you're doing it. Pray. God is listening, even when we don't see an answer right away. Some friends may appreciate a card letting them know they are in your thoughts and prayers.

---

"Make this your common practice: Confess your sins to each other and pray for each other so that you can live together whole and healed. The prayer of a person living right with God is something powerful to be reckoned with."
(James 5:19, The Message Bible)

---

Other Resources for Encouragement

- http://www.nami.org/Find-Support/Family-Members-and-Caregivers
- http://www.mentalhealthministries.net/resources/brochures/scriptures_for_comfort/scripture_comfort.pdf

Essays on Mental Illness

# Appendix II – Resources

National Resources

- National Suicide Prevention Lifeline: 1-800-273-8255
- National Association of Mental Illness (NAMI) https://www.nami.org
- Mental Health America (MHA) www.mentalhealthamerica.net
- The National Institute of Mental Health https://www.nimh.nih.gov

# About the Author

Caroline S. Cooper is an award-winning author and speaker. She is the founder and director of In God's Corner Ministry. Her personal mission is to offer encouragement for life in this complicated world.

One of Caroline's greatest passions is mental health awareness. She is a Missouri certified peer specialist and previously worked for a behavioral health organization. Caroline is an experienced speaker on mental health topics and has presented at the Missouri Department of Mental Health Spring Training Institute as well as the Real Voices, Real Choices conference.

Caroline is a member of the Heart of America Christian Writers Network (HACWN) in Kansas City, Missouri and was selected as their 2017 Writer of the Year. For more than 20 years, she has developed and taught Bible studies for Sunday School and other small groups. She also enjoys preparing unique and interactive presentations on a variety of topics.

Caroline has a Master's in Theology from Calvary Theological Seminary in Kansas City, Missouri, and a Bachelor's in Music Education from the University of Texas-Arlington.

In 1983, Caroline married her college sweetheart, Harry. They have four grown children and two grandchildren. Caroline and Harry live in Lee's Summit, Missouri.

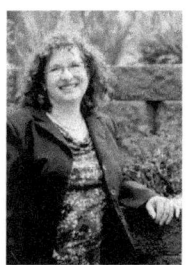

Caroline S. Cooper
410 SE Brentwood Drive
Lee's Summit, MO 64063
(816) 589-0356
caroline@carolinescooper.com
www.carolinescooper.com

www.ingramcontent.com/pod-product-compliance
Lightning Source LLC
Chambersburg PA
CBHW070202230526
45471CB00002B/788